Y0-CDA-586

3rd Edition

Emergency Removal of Patients and First Aid Fire Fighting In Hospitals

by Lt. Robert McGrath

FLORIDA HOSPITAL COLLEGE OF
HEALTH SCIENCES LIBRARY
800 LAKE ESTELLE DRIVE
ORLANDO, FL 32803

21879

**A Joint Publication
of
NATIONAL SAFETY COUNCIL
and
AMERICAN HOSPITAL ASSOCIATION**

WX
185
.E53
1974

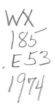

COPYRIGHT© 1956, 1972, AND 1974
BY NATIONAL SAFETY COUNCIL
ALL RIGHTS RESERVED

*No portion of this book may be reproduced by
any process without written permission of the
National Safety Council, 425 North Michigan
Avenue, Chicago, Ill. 60611.*

International Standard Book
Number: O-87912-101-7

Acknowledgments

The information in this manual was gathered through the cooperation and assistance of the American Hospital Association's Council on Hospital Planning and Plant Operations, by the American Hospital Association's Committee on Safety, and its Committee on Disaster Planning.

Appreciation is also expressed to the following hospitals, their officials, and nurses who participated in the development of this manual:

Donna Bonakowski, Karen Weber, Virginia Storey, Emily May, Sandra Potter, Marilyn Brown, Janice DeSanto, Marcia Munton, Teresa Lamkins, MaryAnn Fitzpatrick, and Roosevelt Gallion, L.P.N. (Mount Sinai Hospital Medical Center and I. J. Goldberg School of Nursing).

Miner Brown (Marlborough Hospital), Robert Daly (Hartford Hospital), Jerald Myers (Fort Bayard Medical Center), Raymond Page (Leila Y. Post Montgomery Hospital).

All members of the National Safety Council's Hospital—Health Care Section Fire Safety Committee.

George Pierce (Director of Safety, Little Company of Mary Hospital) and Hyman Levine (Fire Marshal, Mount Sinai Hospital Medical Center).

Paul Seidlitz (St. Elizabeth's Hospital, Chicago) supervised the production of the 15 new photographs used in this Third Edition. The following nurses are pictured: Marsha Davis, Louise Esquival, Janet Everhart, Delores Hillmer, Danuta Kwapisz, and Ellen Trojan.

Special appreciation is also expressed to Fire Commissioner Robert Quinn, and Captain George Arnold of the Chicago Fire Department, who gave their support to Lieutenant McGrath in the development of this manual.

Foreword

The following procedures are techniques for the emergency removal of patients and first aid fire fighting in hospitals.

The techniques described in this manual are a result of Lieutenant Robert McGrath's observations while visiting hospitals in his capacity of Fire Inspector, Chicago Fire Department. He discovered that all nurses knew that in case of fire, patients in immediate danger were to be removed. However, the majority of nurses did not know what proper procedures were to be carried out. He further discovered that he could not tell them how, because an emergency situation in a hospital is vastly different from a like situation in other types of occupancy. Many of the people to be rescued are post-operative cases, or are in casts or traction, or the nature of their illness requires special handling.

The Lieutenant then gathered a group of nurses and together they developed a series of basic carries that were adaptable to patients in various conditions. His most gratifying discovery was that nurses really *want* to know how to react in any emergency. They lent themselves willingly and industriously to the training program that developed from the first labored efforts.

Lieutenant McGrath died in the summer of 1973. Harry A. Pate of McGrath & Pate Associates, Trenton, Mich., is carrying on his work and is responsible for revising the Emergency Removal of Patients portion of this Third Edition.

This booklet is intended as resource material for the hospital safety director, training director, or equivalent. It is not intended as a student instruction manual.

Contents

Introduction

A fire or similar emergency on hospital premises demands instant countermeasures. Effective action at the incipient stage will almost always ensure protection of life and property. Inaction or inadequate measures during the crucial early moments can spell tragic loss to patients, personnel, and plant.

The key to effective action in hospital emergencies is *Training . . . Training of Personnel to Initiate Countermeasures Immediately at the Scene of Threat.*

Such training must aim at developing proficiency in the performance of three main maneuvers—so that all can be started *before* the arrival of a professional fire fighting or disaster-relief team. In a case of fire, these basic actions may be described by the injunctions "Remove Patient," "Fight Fire," and "Start Evacuation."

Along with training of hospital personnel in such basic emergency measures is the need to familiarize them with certain details of hospital building construction, occupancy, and simple fire fighting equipment.

It is intended that this manual will provide an outline and core of information found to be urgently needed in meeting emergencies that can occur in hospitals.

Fire departments of various communities are particularly interested in personnel activity during the few minutes after a fire is discovered and before the first fire company puts in an appearance. Most hospitals have issued written instructions that direct the alerting of many departments and people at the outset of an emergency, but some instructions have not stressed the fact that five minutes is often the deadline between containment and catastrophe. It is with the training of personnel for effective action during those first few minutes that this manual is concerned.

Although the material is directed primarily to nurses and deals with situations likely to be encountered in patient areas, it is pertinent to the duties of every member of the hospital staff and is applicable to every hospital area. In its discussion of emergency training, the content bears on life protection not only in cases of fire and other peacetime dangers, but also in cases of possible wartime eventualities.

1

It is to be emphasized that techniques for "Emergency Removal of Patients" should not be considered detached from the other two main training disciplines set forth. Rather, the three procedures of emergency action should be considered as equally essential and interrelated sequences of a total routine to be followed in the face of peril. Removal of patients from the area of a fire or other hazard is vitally important, but so also is quick extinguishment of the yet small fire and, failing this, starting of evacuation. Therefore, the term: "first aid and fire fighting," which was carefully chosen as a portion for the title of this manual, is first aid given by layman until well-qualified personnel can give assistance that is usually beyond the capabilities of the layman; and fire fighting which is checking the spread of a fire until the fire department arrives, and can professionally control the situation.

PART 1
EMERGENCY REMOVAL
OF PATIENTS

Emergency Removal of Patients

In a hospital fire, the first duty of personnel is to remove the patient or patients who may be in immediate danger. This may require moving one person or many. If eight out of twenty-five patients are helpless (a not unusual proportion), personnel must be trained in workable methods of removing them. Care and treatment of the ill and injured, the new-born, and the aged must also include basic preparedness to cope with unexpected situations. Responsibility for the helpless never ceases.

CARRIES—TECHNIQUES OF IMMEDIATE RESCUE

In the search for the answers to the problem of moving helpless patients, it was found that nurses can handle any of the following removals: (a) carrying patients on stairs and fire escapes; (b) making their own stretchers of blankets and poles; and (c) competently wielding charged hose lines. In two one-hour training sessions, nurses were found to understand completely the full program that is outlined in this manual. With one additional hour of training, they were competent to instruct others.

Several factors must be considered in emergency handling of patients: (a) the nature of the emergency; (b) the weight and condition of the patient; and (c) the strength and adaptability of the rescuer. Of the carries to be discussed, opinions vary as to which technique is the easiest for a person to perform. *Each person must find the one carry that he or she can handle best.* If a person practices the carry often enough, the patient's weight and height will not become important factors.

Another factor is the height of the bed. Patients in variable height beds in the "low" position and in low beds should be removed with the one-, two-, or three-man cradle or kneel drop to a blanket, described in the following pages.

On all carries, patients must be "hugged" firmly. The carrier should use his own body and that of the patient to sustain the patient's weight. These removals are designed for distribution of a patient's weight over the whole of the carrier's body, rather

5

than for its concentration on his hands and arms alone. When one carries a heavy bag or package, he does not transport it with his arms extended full length from his body. He "hugs" the object to his side where the process is then part "lift" and part "press" with a degree of frictional assistance from the object against body resistance. Often in carrying groceries, for example, a person will take his hands away from the bottom of the bag entirely and support the weight by hugging the middle of the bag so that it is really suspended between the pressure of his body and the pressure of his arms.

Basically there are only five removals or carries: the hip carry for one nurse, the cradle drop for one nurse, the extremity carry for two nurses, the swing carry for two nurses, and the three-man carry for three nurses. The rest are variations of these depending upon the personnel available and the weight and condition of the patient.

———————

CARRIES FOR ONE NURSE

HIP CARRY

If the nurse approaches from the patient's right side, she pulls the patient's left arm over her left shoulder by grasping the patient's left wrist with her left hand, palm down. She pulls down on the arm, raising and turning the patient's body so she can slide her right hand into the right armpit. (The procedure is reversed if the nurse approaches from the patient's left.)

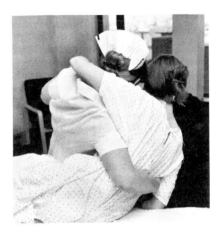

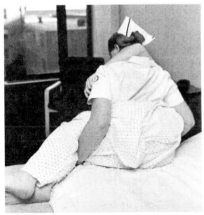

The nurse then releases the patient's wrist, makes a half turn to her left so that her hips are squarely against the patient's abdomen. With her knees slightly bent and her feet apart, she reaches back with her left arm and grasps both of the knees. Now she has the patient secured by the armpit and the knees.

7

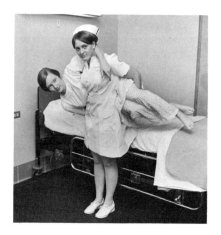

The nurse draws the patient up on her hips before she leaves the bedside. If she carries the patient on her buttocks, the patient may start to slide. A great deal of the lifting power results from the nurse pushing against the floor with her feet as she stands as erectly as possible and straightens her knees. She walks with her chest out and her shoulders back.

To unload the patient in the corridor, the nurse places the patient's buttocks against the wall and drops on her knee closer to the wall. Leaning against the patient as the person slides down the wall, the nurse uses the wall to sustain the patient's weight and to maintain her own balance. The patient is locked between her body and the wall.

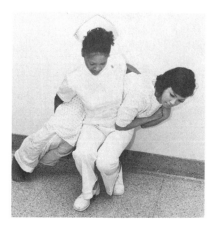

8

THE SLIDE OR CRADLE DROP

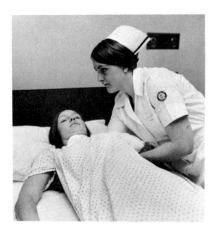

First, the nurse doubles a blanket lengthwise and places it on the floor, parallel to and next to the bed.

She then stands next to the bed. Her knee (or thigh) that is nearer the head of the bed is placed against the bed, opposite the patient's shoulders. Both feet are flat on the floor, about six inches apart, with the foot farther from the head being about six inches from the bed.

The nurse slips her hand that is nearer the head of the bed under the patient's neck and continues until she grasps the patient's far shoulder and the patient's head rests on her arm.

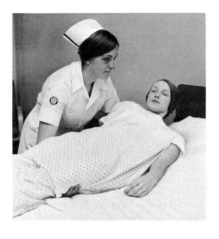

She slips her other arm under the patient's knees and grasps the far leg.

The nurse does not lift the patient but, rather, pulls with both hands while pushing against the bed with her knee (or thigh).

The relative position of the patient's body is important. The nurse cannot maintain her balance if she pulls the patient's·buttocks from the bed first. The order in which to move the patient from the bed is first the ankles; then the knees, thighs, buttocks, and chest; and finally the shoulders and head.

9

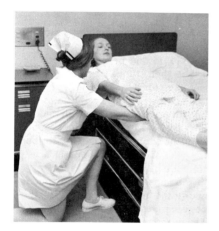

The moment that the patient starts to leave the bed, the nurse drops to her knee further from the head of the bed.

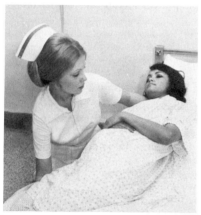

As the patient clears the bed, the nurse's arm that is under the patient's knees controls the lower portion of the patient. The cradle formed by the knee and arms protects the patient's back.

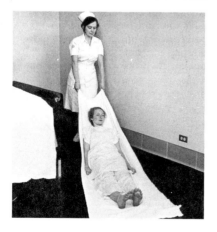

The nurse lets the patient slide gently to the blanket. She then pulls the blanket and the patient from the room, head first.

10

THE PACK-STRAP CARRY

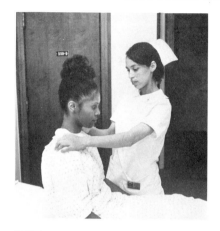

The nurse brings the patient to a sitting position by elevating the back rest (if time permits) or by pulling the patient to a sitting position. She grasps each wrist.

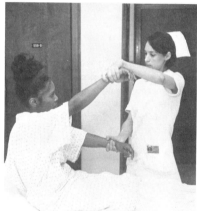

The nurse takes a step backwards with the leg nearer the head of the bed. She raises the wrist that is further from her and turns herself. She slips under the raised arm and places her back squarely against the patient's chest.

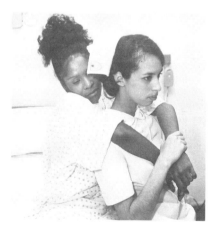

The nurse then pulls the patient's arms over her shoulders and crosses them on her own chest.

11

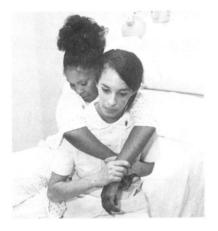

The nurse pulls downward on the arms and leans slightly forward, bending her shoulders only.

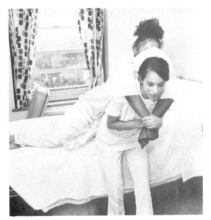

The nurse turns both her body and her feet sharply around toward the head of the bed. It is not necessary to drag or lift the patient—the forward momentum of this turn should roll the patient on to the nurse's back easily.

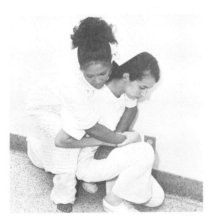

To unload the patient, the nurse leans the patient's shoulder against a wall and also leans against the patient. She drops to her knee closer to the wall and lowers both herself and the patient. She can ease the patient to the floor by allowing the patient to roll off her shoulder and hip. The patient will be secure between the wall and the nurse's body.

ANKLE ROLL

If a nurse finds a patient lying on the floor, she places a blanket, open to full length, parallel to the body. She then places the arm closest to the blanket down the side of the body. For purposes of the removal, it makes no difference if the patient is face down or face up.

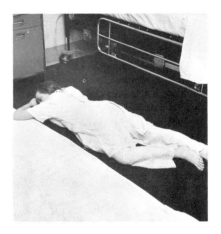

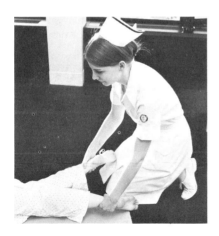

The nurse takes the ankle that is farther from the blanket and places it on top of the nearer ankle. She keeps her back rigid and uses her arms to press down on the top ankle and pull up on the bottom ankle in order to turn the patient over on to the blanket. She pulls the blanket and the patient head first from the room.

HIP ROLL

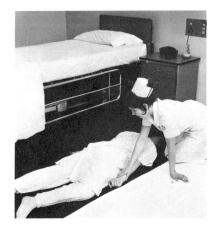
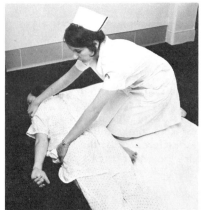

A variation of the ankle roll is the use of the shoulder and hip bone as pulling points. This method is probably easier in most instances and should always be used if the patient is very heavy or has injuries which preclude the use of the ankle roll.

The nurse places the patient's arm by the side next to the blanket and then drops to one knee on the blanket just above the patient's hips. Her other foot is flat on the blanket. She leans forward and grasps the patient by the far shoulder and hip bone and rolls the patient over toward her with a steady pull, moving back out of the way as she does so.

On all blanket drags, the blanket must extend six or eight inches beyond the head to avoid injury. If the patient's feet are closer to the door, the nurse must spin the blanket and pull the patient out, head foremost.

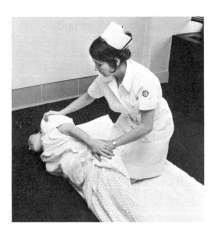
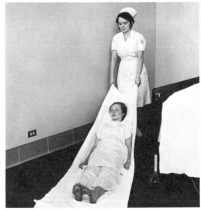

CARRIES FOR TWO NURSES

SWING CARRY

If the nurses approach from the patient's left, the first nurse, standing with her feet together, slips her right arm under the patient's neck and grasps the right shoulder in her right hand. She slides her left palm behind the left biceps and grips the patient's upper left arm. She brings the patient to a sitting position by taking one step with the left foot toward the foot of the bed. This

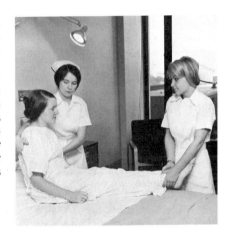

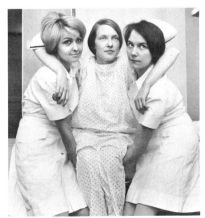

move employs the swing of her whole body. She gains additional leverage if she pushes her right shoulder against the patient's left shoulder once the patient is in motion. When the patient is sitting, the second nurse grasps the ankles and swings the feet off the bed. (If the nurses approach from the right, all the mechanics are reversed.)

Both nurses stand close to the patient's side, facing in the same direction. Each takes one of the patient's wrists and pulls the arm around her neck and down across her chest. Each nurse then reaches across the patient's back and places her free hand on the top of the other nurse's shoulder.

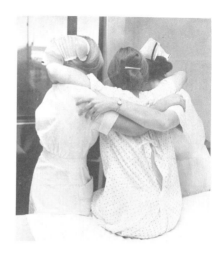

Both nurses then release the patient's wrists. Each reaches under the patient's knees and grasps the wrist of the other nurse. If the nurse at the right side reaches under with her right palm down, and the nurse at the left side reaches under with her left palm up, their hands will quickly lock together.

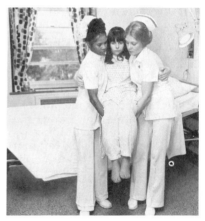

The patient is removed from the bed by both nurses pushing up with their shoulders. Weight makes no material difference because the patient is hanging like a pendulum off the nurse's shoulders. This is the easiest removal of all, and is the two-man carry used on stairs and fire escapes. Any two nurses can carry any patient anywhere.

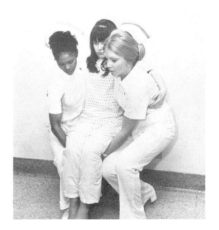

To unload in the corridor, each nurse drops on the knee closer to the patient. While leaning against the patient, the nurses place the individual's buttocks on the floor, and lower the patient to her back.

16

EXTREMITY
CARRY

The first nurse brings the patient to a sitting position in the same manner described in the swing carry. When the patient is sitting, she places her arms through the armpits and grips her own wrist above the patient's chest. The second nurse approaches from the same side and halts at the patient's feet. With her left hand under the patient's left heel, she pulls the left ankle clear of the bed as she slides between the patient's legs as far as the patient's right knee.

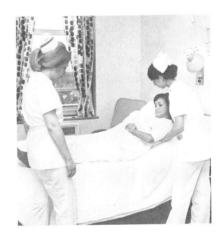

As the second nurse makes a half turn left, she grasps the patient's right knee under her right arm. Completing the turn, she transfers her left hand to the patient's left knee, which she then encircles with her left arm. She now has a leg under each arm.

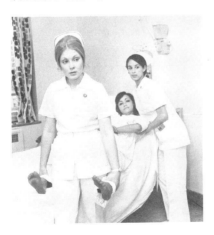

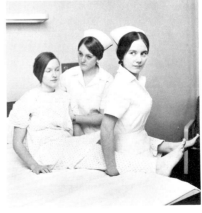

Both nurses then take one step away from the bed and carry the patient from the room. Like so many other carries, this involves a "hugging" action, with the patient's back carried tight against the first nurse's chest, the patient's shoulders as close to the level of hers as possible.

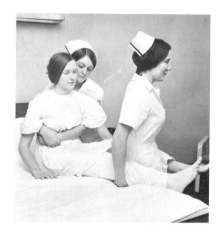

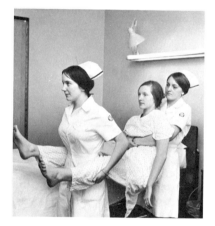

To unload the patient in the corridor, the second nurse stoops with her right foot slightly behind and about six inches from her left and lowers the patient's legs to the floor. The first nurse lets the patient slide down her body until the buttocks reach the

floor. Then she lowers the patient to his back. This is a very fast removal. (Any two nurses can carry any patient. The carry is useful when the path of exit is narrow because of furniture or fire.)

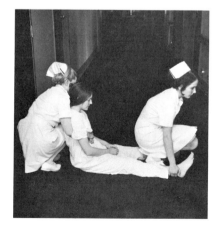

DOUBLE
CRADLE DROP

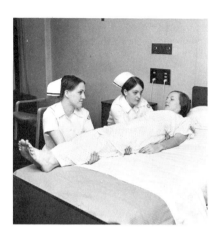

The nurses place a blanket, folded lengthwise, on the floor next to the bed.

They stand next to the bed, one opposite the patient's shoulders and the other opposite the knees. The nurses kneel on the knee closer to the center of the bed. They place the knee (or thigh) nearer the head (or the foot) of the bed against the bed.

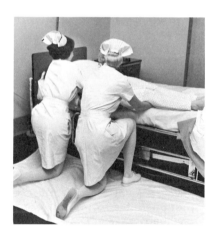

The nurse nearer the head of the bed slips one hand under the patient's neck and grasps the far shoulder. She grasps the biceps of the patient's near arm with her other hand.

The other nurse grips the patient's legs—one hand is placed above the knee; the other, below.

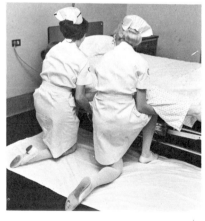

Both nurses push against the bed with their knees (thighs) and pull the patient toward them. The nurses pull the patient off the bed and against their chests, drop their extended knees to the floor, and slide the patient gently down to the blanket.

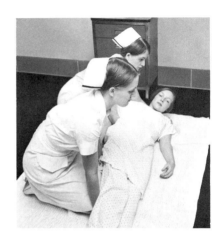

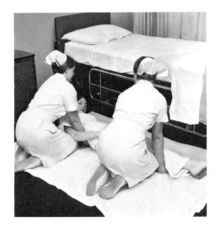

This type of removal has an advantage over the extended knee removal for a fracture or post-operative case, for example; because there may be less risk of aggravating the injury by use of a body slide instead of a knee removal.

CARRIES FOR THREE NURSES

THREE-MAN CARRY

The first nurse slips her arm under the patient's neck and grasps the patient's far shoulder in her hand. She slips her other hand under the small of the patient's back, as far as it will go. The second nurse slips both arms under the patient's body, one above the buttocks and one below, reaching under as far as possible. The third nurse slips both arms under the patient's legs and grips them above and below the knees. (It is desirable

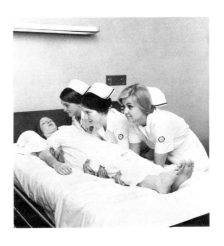

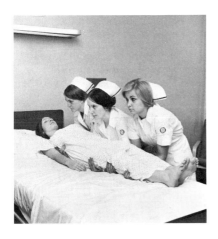

for the tallest nurse to take the shoulder position because that is the key point in turning the patient.)

The nurses slide the patient to the edge of the bed, lift together and turn the patient to face them, and then carry the individual on their chests. The "slide" is very important, because it greatly simplifies the lifting. The "slide" and "lift" should be a continuous action.

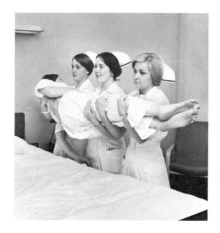

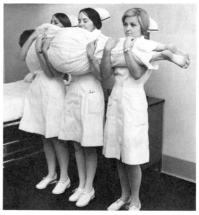

When leaving the room, the nurses swing out with the patient's feet first. They go through the doorway obliquely—that is, in a staggered single file. This line-up allows each nurse about four or five inches of floor space for fast and safe walking.

If the patient is not too heavy, the three nurses can drop on the knee closer to the patient's feet and lower the individual, first to their knees, and then to the floor by withdrawing their extended knees.

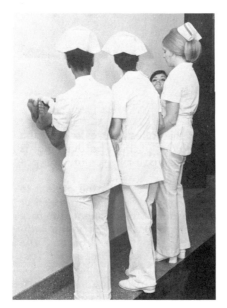

If the patient is quite heavy and a fourth nurse is not handy, the three nurses should face the corridor wall, place the patient's body against the wall and let it slide down, first to their knees and then to the floor. If the nurses lean against the patient, the wall will bear most of the weight.

CARRIES FOR
FOUR NURSES

FOUR-MAN
BLANKET CARRY

Use the three-man carry to lower the patient to the floor next to a blanket doubled lengthwise.

If four nurses are available for carrying, one squats at each of the patient's shoulders and at each of the patient's knees. Those at the shoulders grip the blanket above the

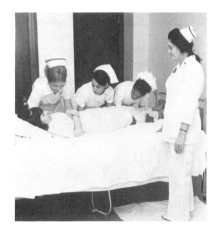

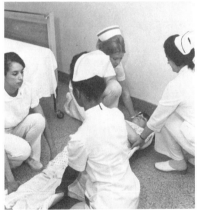

shoulders and opposite the elbows. Those at the knees grip the blanket six inches above and six inches below the patient's knees. They roll the blanket toward the patient, with the palms of their hands down, until their knuckles are tight against the patient's body.

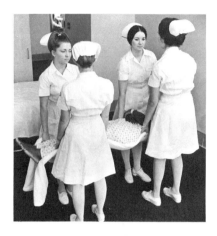 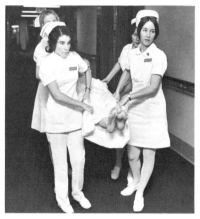

All the nurses lift together; they keep their backs straight and lift with their legs. Arms are extended.

The bearers must carry with their hands hip high, not at arm's length. Down a hallway, stairway, or fire escape, the patient is moved feet first.

ADDITIONAL CARRIES FOR THREE NURSES

Several additional carries differ from those illustrated only in details and in the number of nurses used.

One is the three-man bed to wheeled stretcher carry. When using wheeled stretchers in conjunction with the three-man bed removal, best results are obtained by placing the wheeled stretcher at right angles at the foot of the bed. The three nurses slide the patient to the edge of the bed, and then lift and turn him so that he is carried on the chests of all three. The nurse at the feet of the patient then steps backward in a wide arc from the bed; the second nurse makes a smaller swing back, and the nurse at the head has only to turn 90 degrees; then all three walk forward together to the stretcher. If at times this is not feasible, the wheeled stretcher can be right-angled at the head of the bed, or placed parallel to the side of the bed. The latter position requires a complete swing around by two carriers standing between the bed and stretcher, and rather than do this, it might be better to place the head of the wheeled stretcher against the foot of the bed, so that the nurses can walk straight ahead to the cart in a slightly oblique manner. A third nurse should assist by standing at the opposite side of the cart.

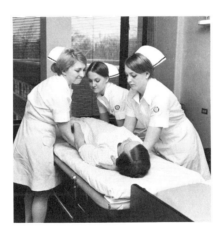

A nonwheeled stretcher or blanket, as well as a wheeled stretcher, can be placed at right angles at the foot of the bed. Again, as mentioned above, the three nurses slide the patient to the edge of the bed, lift and turn him so that he is carried on the chests of all three, and then swing back in an arc so that they can approach the stretcher or blanket abreast. After reaching the stretcher, they drop on one knee and lower the patient to their knee level and finally to the stretcher or blanket. When three nurses carry a nonwheeled stretcher, two should be at the head and the third at the foot where there is less weight. All should face the direction of intended travel even if this requires swinging the stretcher about. The first two bearers carry the stretcher with one hand, the third uses both hands.

The triple cradle drop and the triple knee drop are identical with the two-man cradle and two-man kneel drops, except that a third nurse takes a position between the first two and assists in pulling the patient out on their knees or chests. At the start, the third nurse slips one hand above the patient's buttocks and one hand below. When the patient is on the blanket, he can be easily turned in any direction. If the head of the bed is against the wall and opposite the door, this presents no problem because when the head of the blanket is turned about, the patient's body and legs will pivot under the bed.

Evacuation of Patients

Evacuation of patients and personnel *out of the hospital building* should be a last resort. Hospital evacuation is an entirely different process than that recommended for schools and factories. In the latter establishments, the objective is to clear the building in three minutes.

In a hospital, a third of the patients are assumed to be helpless, with many others in various degrees of dependency. Another obstacle to outside retreat is the general state of patient undress.

Familiarity with the tactics of patient evacuation is a necessity in any hospital. Because of the differences in structural design of buildings, a plan that may suit one hospital may not suit another. Evacuation can be either horizontal or vertical movement from a dangerous or potentially dangerous area to one of comparative safety.

Actual tests have shown that quick removals by bed or mattress from a room in a fire emergency are not practical even at best and are often impossible. There is no merit in a mattress removal under any condition. Patients should be removed from burning rooms by either a carry or a blanket drag. After the patients have been removed from immediate danger, an attempt must be made to subdue the fire with extinguishers and the hose line. If this is impossible, the door and transom must be closed and the threshold sealed with a wet towel or blanket. The next step is to sound a general alarm and proceed with further removal of patients to the extent necessary. This may involve the total evacuation of the hospital, particularly in cases of conflagration or dense smoke or fumes throughout the building.

HORIZONTAL FLOW

Patients are removed laterally by wheeled stretcher, non-wheeled stretcher, wheelchair, blanket, or other conveyance to the nearest and safest protected area. Patients in immediate danger should be moved first, including those who might be separated from safety, if the fire enters the corridor. Next to move (contrary to some opinion) should be the ambulatory patients. Panic is less likely to be caused by helpless people. Those who are ambulatory should be instructed to line up outside their rooms; form a chain by holding hands; and follow a lead nurse into a safe area. The rooms should be checked for stragglers and all windows and doors closed when the rooms are vacated. The patients should be rechecked in the refuge. When horizontal evacuation is ordered, the personnel in the receiving area should assist in the removal. If there are fire doors, they should be closed. If there are smoke barriers, the thresholds should be sealed. Engineering should shut off all ventilation immediately. Finally, all personnel should remain alert for any further movement.

VERTICAL FLOW

Vertical or downward movement to a safe area is used if corridor separation is lacking on the floor involved in the fire. If stairwells and shafts are enclosed, refuge can be found on one floor below the fire, but two is recommended, if time permits. Ambulatory patients should again form a chain and follow a lead nurse.

Under "normal" emergency conditions elevators should never be used in the actual fire wing at any time. In a central bank complex, or in remote locations, elevators should also not be used unless declared safe by the responsible fire or hospital authority at the scene. If possible, the elevators should be brought to the first floor and held there on MANUAL to await the arrival of the fire department, who may use them, if they are usable.

A written or implied order like NEVER USE THE ELEVATORS could turn into a death order in *any* type of high-rise construction. If conditions are such that you *have* to use an elevator, those techniques involving the use of blankets are best for loading and unloading helpless carry cases. The best stairway or fire escape carries are the two-man swing carry and the three-man and four-man blanket carries.

If there are enclosed stairwells at corridor extremities, but an open well or rotunda in the center, then the safe terminal may well be in the basement. Where there are open wells, shafts, and chutes throughout, vertical evacuation of all floors must be considered. This may require first moving horizontally to a stairwell temporarily remote from the smoke and fire, or limiting the evacuation to the most remote fire escapes. In structures of this type, the next acute area of danger is the very top floor. A place of safety might mean the basement, another building, or an area considerably removed from the hospital.

To prepare for evacuation of any kind, particularly vertical and total, personnel should be trained to perform certain duties as teams or units. In case of disaster, there will then be a competent army to perform automatically. There should be LOADING teams to get patients on wheeled stretchers, wheelchairs, nonwheeled stretchers, and blankets. There should also be MOVING teams to get these conveyances to the elevators and stairways; and CARRYING teams to get the patients down stairs and fire escapes. These practically-trained people could be called "loaders," "movers," and "carriers." This is a more orderly arrangement than having single teams tackle three phases.

EVACUATION EQUIPMENT

Wheeled stretchers and wheelchairs

A wheeled stretcher is loaded by using the three-man carry; a wheelchair with the swing carry. Both conveyances can be pushed onto elevators, usually two wheeled stretchers or three or four wheelchairs, depending upon the size of the elevator. When the wheeled stretcher and wheelchairs are used to bring patients to a stairway or fire escape, patients are taken off and carried with the two-man swing carry in both cases. When emptied, these devices are taken back to the emergency area for use with other patients.

Blankets

Of all the possible equipment that can be used for evacuation, the blanket is more important than any other. It can be used to smother fire, or to drag a patient from a room. It can be made into a stretcher, with or without poles, for carrying patients in halls, on stairs, or fire escapes. It may be possible to remove six or eight patients on blankets in the same time it might take two nurses to steer a bed out of a room.

When the blanket is doubled lengthwise for use as a stretcher, patients can be carried by three or four nurses. One, two, or three nurses can place the patient on the blanket.

Actually, for vertical evacuation there is a choice of four removals, depending upon the personnel available, condition of the patient, and other factors. The two-man swing carry, the three-man and four-man blanket carry, and the pole-and-blanket stretcher carry can all be used.

Blanket stretchers

Nonwheeled stretchers are of great value in any disaster planning, but such stretchers are rare in most hospitals for several reasons, one of which is the problem of storage. Where nonwheeled stretchers are available, or not enough such stretchers provided, the personnel can improvise these devices by the use of poles and blankets. There are plenty of blankets available and the poles can be purchased at low cost. The poles must be six-feet long and one and five-eighths inches in diameter in soft wood, or one and one-fourth inches in diameter in hardwood.

To assemble the blanket and poles, the blanket is spread on the floor and the first pole placed across the width of the blanket, about in the center. One edge of the blanket is pulled over to about ten inches from the opposite edge. With the two edges of the blanket parallel to each other but ten inches apart, the second pole is placed eight-inches inside the top edge. Then the bottom edge is pulled all the way over to the first pole. One nurse can make a blanket stretcher, but it is easier and faster for two. Two, three, or four nurses can carry it.

A good nonwheeled stretcher carry is the four-man shoulder carry. Personnel can carry more weight for longer distances on their shoulders than in their hands. Four nurses can bring the patient and stretcher from the floor to their shoulders. To do this, each nurse takes a corner position at the side of the stretcher and faces the nurse opposite her. All reach down with palms up and grasp the pole near the end with one hand, and toward the center with the other hand. At command, the stretcher is lifted waist high and then pushed shoulder high in one continuous sweep. When the stretcher is at shoulder height, all four nurses turn and face the direction of travel, placing their shoulders under the pole.

If for any reason it is necessary to change the direction, this can be accomplished easily by all four nurses doing an about-face, pivoting toward the patient and placing the other shoulder under the pole, rather than attempting to swing the patient and the stretcher. Nurses have carried patients up stairs as well as down on these improvised stretchers. To set the stretcher in a safe area, the nurses again must put both hands on the pole, face each other, and lower the stretcher first to arm's length, and then to the floor. The poles can be pulled out and taken back to the emergency area for further use.

SPECIAL PROBLEMS

Evacuation of infants

A major problem in any hospital is the evacuation of infants. Hospitals may have thirty or forty or eighty infants, who may have to be moved to a safe area. The advice that each mother be given only her own baby is sentimental but not too practical. Under

30

smoke conditions it is often impossible to tell one end of a baby from the other. Firemen remove babies as quickly as possible without establishing their identity and without assistance from people who are naturally frightened.

It has been proposed that four or five bassinets be lined up across the corridor so that one nurse can wheel them away. This might work if the horizontal exit is wide enough, and if bassinets could be pushed easily. Frequently they cannot be. However, it should not be forgotten that horizontal evacuation may be just the initial step in a series of retreating movements, particularly in the absence of area separations. Crowding thirty or forty wheeled bassinets around a stairwell might eliminate the chance of vertical evacuation for the babies or anyone else, to say nothing of the hampering effect on fire fighting.

Here again the blanket is the most important implement to consider. Babies are hardier little creatures than is usually supposed. A number of them can be dragged or carried on a blanket without injury. Then, any method or avenue of retreat can be used.

Using this removal provides an opportunity to employ calm mothers. It can be explained that all the babies will be saved if they cooperate. If one can show the mothers that each blanket will handle twelve or fourteen babies, the mothers will understand. If two nurses can carry a 200-pound man down a stairway, then 140 pounds of babies is not a carrying problem for two or more nurses.

Evacuation of children

Children can be handled like other patients except that in ambulatory evacuation it might be advisable to alternate the older and younger children in the evacuation line. Where only two nurses are available, the important posts are at the front and at the end of the line. Someone has to lead the way and someone has to be responsible that no one is left behind.

Evacuation of psychiatric patients

In general hospitals having a psychiatric ward or section, there are usually specially trained personnel assigned to the care of these patients. In any emergency entailing movement of such patients, it is desirable that their regularly assigned personnel handle the evacuation.

In handling psychiatric patients, nurses and doctors state that they anticipate no greater difficulty than is usually met in handling children. Only a small percentage of mental patients is likely to be violent, and even this small number would not necessarily cause trouble in a fire; but the possibility must be considered. Mental patients can best be controlled and accounted for by everyone using the same exit in an evacuation.

———————

PART 2
FIRST AID FIRE FIGHTING IN HOSPITALS

First Aid Fire Fighting in Hospitals

PREPAREDNESS

Fire fighting begins with fire prevention and fire safety. Fire safety depends, in part, upon the sensible and practical provision of structural protection, occupancy isolation, and proper distribution of hospital fire fighting equipment. The foremost consideration of any institution must be the safety of its occupants, regardless of minimum or maximum code interpretation by either national, state, or local authorities, or insurance carriers. It is not the purpose of this manual to detail a complete fire prevention program, but a certain amount of background material is necessary for everyone who must be prepared to deal with fire emergencies.

Structure

Many persons consider that brick, concrete, or steel construction will create a fireproof hospital. This opinion is not justifiable when one considers that boiler rooms, kitchens, laundries, maintenance shops, laboratories, pharmacies, and operating rooms are all grouped under one roof. These potential hazards exist even in a well constructed building.

No building has been designed that can be termed fire-proof. A modern structure may be fire-resistant, but not fire-proof. Resistance is provided by steel and concrete construction, but even steel must be encased in concrete or other heat-resistant material to prevent buckling and collapsing from extremely high temperatures.

A new fire-resistant building is comparable to a new furnace. If nothing is put into the furnace, there can be no fire in it. If paper, wood, coal, or oil is introduced into a furnace, or if furniture and other combustible equipment, or flammable liquids and gases are introduced into a fire-resistant building, the fire potentialities can be identical. All that is needed is a source of ignition. One match or one spark may be sufficient. Once started, the fire will continue to burn in both the furnace and the fire-resistant building until the fuel is exhausted or the fire extinguished.

Relative to the structure of a building, other fire-resistive precautions include the enclosure of vertical openings and the installation of fire doors and corridor separations. Normally fire races up vertical openings and the resulting pressure will cause horizontal spread of the fire. The roofs and floors of fire-resistant buildings are fire resistive. Therefore, the spread of heat and fire may be horizontal and then downward, unless successfully confined to the immediate area of origin. Fire doors and corridor separations are intended to check such horizontal spread.

In answer to an often asked question regarding the absence of outside fire escapes on many modern high-structure hospitals, it should be pointed out that every enclosed stairwell is a fire escape. The very first step in hospital security, should be to enclose all vertical openings to retard the normal upward sweep of smoke and heat. The doors to these potential fire flues should be approved metal or metal-clad doors, be self-closing, and should never be wedged open. Transoms over doors on stairwells should be eliminated or permanently secured and protected. A stairwell properly enclosed is both a refuge and a route to safety. Elevator shafts, trash chutes, dumb waiters, and pipe chases are other passages that require protection against vertical fire spread. All windows in the immediate vicinity of an exterior fire escape should be made of wired glass.

Regardless of whether floor areas are fifteen hundred or fifteen thousand square feet, they should be separated into at least two fire sections to facilitate horizontal evacuation. If a building has firewalls bisecting it, an approved fire door should be installed on each side of each wall opening. If a building is fire-resistant, smoke barriers should be installed in the corridors to ensure safe areas to which retreats can be made.

Occupancy

There are many locations and procedures in a hospital which are hazardous, yet are indispensable. Liberal provision of fire doors with fusible links, sprinkler heads, explosion-proof fittings and vapor-proof globes, vents, fall-out windows and raised door sills on vaults where flammable liquids are stored, automatic alarms, and correct extinguishers have proven to be of value in confining a fire to its original area. For example, there is no reason why a paint shop fire should involve the carpenter shop, the electric shop, or the plumbing shop if each of these rooms is properly isolated. A basement fire should be confined to that particular area. This is the control phase so important in fire extinguishment. Control installations which can be made in these instances at a relatively small expense can mean the difference between an incipient fire quickly extinguished and a holocaust costing scores of lives and countless dollars.

Equipment

One of the most important aspects of hospital first aid fire fighting is a sensible installation, arrangement, and maintenance of fire fighting equipment. Location of a single fire extinguisher in dead center of a 150 foot corridor, for no other reason than to meet the 75 foot walking distance requirement of a code, is a meager and misdirected safety measure. The placement of a soda acid extinguisher in surgery, laboratories, or the pharmacy, where the aqueous content of the extinguisher is apt to spread a fire or cause an explosion, violates a principle of safety. If the proper extinguisher is provided, it should not be located in the interior of the room where it is beyond the reach of someone fleeing toward the door as a natural reaction to sudden or unexpected ignition. The prescribed location for an efficient extinguisher would be on the wall, adjacent to a doorway, on either side.

Perhaps the best method of equipment placement is the grouping together of a fire alarm, extinguishers, and a hose line in a compact fire station near an enclosed stairwell. The equipment should be installed at identical locations on each floor from basement to roof. Instead of a person having to look one place for the extinguisher; a second place for the alarm; and a third place for the hose; it is easier for him to associate all equipment with one specific station. This is doubly important in the interfloor response which will be discussed later. Each such location should always be referred to as the fire station. In some hospitals, this arrangement may not be feasible, but at least an extinguisher should be placed next to an alarm box or telephone so that the person turning in the alarm can immediately return with a firefighting weapon. No one is more likely to know where the extinguisher is needed than the person who turns in the alarm. (Some hospitals have two or more fire stations on each floor.)

Personnel

Protective procedures before the arrival of the fire department depends on the immediate coordinated response of trained people. A fire which does not receive the necessary attention in the first five minutes or less can assume serious proportions from then on. Professional firemen either confine or subdue a blaze in that length of time or are forced to call for additional equipment and manpower.

Fighting fire is waging war against smoke, heat, flame, and

whatever panic exists. The degree of panic can usually be measured by the presence or absence of people who know how to react to the unexpected. In addition to the use of specified fire fighting equipment, it is advantageous for hospital personnel to be able to apply a little muscle, courage, and good judgment when and where needed. Training personnel to respond effectively to a fire emergency is the very heart of any fire fighting program. Each person must know exactly what to do and must have enough practice to be able to perform quickly and efficiently. Response to emergencies should be planned. Often hospital fire drills bring in a response of 40 or 50 people which is neither realistic or desirable. It is much better to use four, eight, or twelve people who have had a measure of training. The first four people make the first team, and there is no rule that says these four, and the next four, *have* to be nurses.

HOSPITAL FIRE BRIGADES

Fire brigades composed of employees are used extensively in plants and factories and are important assets because their members have special training in fire fighting; have a knowledge of the property; and, perhaps most important, are available. In hospitals, the constant movement and change of personnel complicates the problem of availability. Although a hospital engineer may start out with ten or twenty men in the morning, by ten o'clock he may find it quite impossible to gather four or five together in less than thirty minutes; and, of course, at least one man must remain on watch in the boiler room. The conditions on evening and night shifts become gradually more acute, and help from the boiler room can only supplement whatever action has already been taken in the threatened area.

Composition

The staff of a small hospital is limited even in the daytime and planning must take this into account. In small hospitals, perhaps more than anywhere else, the adequate training of every member of the staff in emergency techniques is a necessity, for any one of them may be required to handle an emergency situation with little or no help.

In larger hospitals, the three-staff people closest to the fire, plus the switchboard operator and the elevator operator (if the staff includes one) may be designated as a permanent nucleus of a functional fire brigade during daytime. This complement would form a direct line of communication and transportation preliminary to and, later, cooperating with the work of the fire department. (A telephone on the elevator may be an additional advantage.)

Brigade response

Although other staff members will also respond, the following is an example of what can be done in a hospital with five people acting as a nucleus of a fire brigade:

It is early afternoon and there are three nurses in a patient area. The first nurse notices smoke coming from a three-bed room about twenty-feet away. She goes into the room and finds that the fire is coming from a bed near the window. She makes a hip carry removal of the patient from the bed, and then starts for the alarm. The second and third nurses have now seen the smoke. The second nurse brings an extinguisher; the third stretches a hose line to the door of the room. Both remove the next patient closest to the fire with a swing carry. By this time, the first nurse has pulled the alarm and returned with another extinguisher. All three go in and remove the third patient, who has a broken leg, with the three-man carry. The first and second nurses then use their extinguishers on the fire.

By now two beds, the curtains, and the venetian blinds are involved; so the nurses discard the extinguishers, leave the room, and close the door. They pick up the hose nozzle and signal to the third nurse who has gone to the water valve. When the water reaches the nozzle, the two nurses, kneeling on either side of the hose line, push open the door and move the stream up and down and side-to-side, decreasing the intensity of the fire. As they stand up to advance into the room, the engineer and three men from the fire department relieve them of the hose line. The time elapsed since the first nurse saw the smoke is less than three minutes.

When the alarm rang at the switchboard, the operator relayed the information to the fire department. This call went through even though the internal alarm system was connected directly to the fire department. The hospital is large and the operator gave the fire department additional information so that the men could go directly to the location of the fire, preventing any unnecessary delay.

Interfloor response

The foregoing is an example of an ideal response in a hospital. A primary response of this kind need present no particular problem in the daytime. During the night, however, or in a small hospital, only one nurse may be available to an entire floor area.

If a fire occurs, she will need help quickly; and there is no one closer to a lone nurse in trouble than the nurse on the floor above or the nurse on the floor below. Nurses on the floor above and the floor below the fire can be notified quickly in several ways. A code signal on the public address system, a call via the switchboard, a buzzer, or any other convenient and effective system can be used.

If the nurse above walks down ten feet and the nurse below walks up ten feet, they are in a position to form a team with the first nurse who is need of aid. Naturally, if the fire occurs on the bottom floor of the patient area, or the top floor of the patient area, the interfloor response would bring nurses from the two floors above the fire or the two floors below the fire, with relatively little loss of time.

It has been found that a team of three, properly instructed, can cope with almost any emergency in the incipient stage. This "unit-of-three" theory assumes that the first three arrivals constitute an emergency fire brigade in any part of the hospital.

In a public demonstration at a hospital in Chicago, a three-bed "room" was set up in the courtyard and this interfloor response was used. Nurses came from the basement, the first, second, and third floors in various three-man drill combinations. Each drill required carrying three "patients" from their beds into a tunnel located twenty-five feet from the first bed and thirty-five feet from the third bed. Then the first two nurses applied two extinguishers to a small fire near the beds, while the third nurse stretched a hose line and placed it at the feet of the first two. When the third nurse started back toward the water valve, the first two discarded their extinguishers, picked up the hose nozzle, and operated the water stream on a larger fire behind the beds. In these various drills, three "patients" were carried out, two pressure extinguishers were used, and a charged hose line operated in one minute or less. The drills were set in motion by the first nurse activating a portable fire-alarm set up near the tunnel.

An inspection showed that another hospital can assemble twenty-one people at a daytime emergency in less than three minutes. In the middle of the night, however, the positive response was limited to one nurse and one attendant, discounting one more person who might or might not be available from the boiler room, which is seventeen floors below the top patient floor in this particular hospital. The solution to this problem was to introduce the interfloor response. With the nurse and attendant present on the emergency floor, the attendant from above and the attendant from below, a competent team of four was organized . . . a team that could cope adequately with a difficult situation until the arrival of the fire department and other hospital aid.

These suggestions for interfloor response are proposed because it is believed that this is the most effective way to confine the fire to its point of origin and save those in immediate danger. To the objection that nurses should not leave their posts, the answer may be given that one nurse probably could not handle the emergency, and that in a few minutes the lone nurses on the other floors might be in the same predicament. One of the first things a fireman learns is not to undertake a hazardous task alone.

FIRST AID FIRE FIGHTING TECHNIQUES

In addition to specific techniques of patient removal there are specific techniques of fire fighting that should be known and practiced. There should be no uncertainty in bed fires. The rule is to *get the patient on the floor*. In an oxygen tent fire, *first shut off the oxygen, then get the patient on the floor*.

Bed fires

In both situations, if the rescuer has a blanket, he can use it to smother the fire and also as a dragging device. There are cases on record where bed fires became too intense for the rescuer to attempt a removal without protection from flame injury. Keeping in mind that the patient must be taken *out* of the fire, it may be necessary first to drape a blanket over him so that one edge extends to the floor and acts as a shield for the person or persons making the removal.

It is possible in a bed fire to cover the patient with a blanket, and then knead the blanket as one kneads dough until the fire is subdued enough to permit the next necessary steps. (Incidentally, anything that can be done with a blanket can also be done with a sheet.) The fear of handling people who are "on fire" is not warranted.

When a patient is in traction, or is restrained by any other means, and becomes involved in a fire, the implements immediately required are a blanket and a cutting tool. If there is any question of responsibility in removing someone from traction, it should be remembered that there is always a chance of a patient recovering from an aggravated fracture, but never from the logical alternative. The kneel drop for one nurse, the kneel drop for two nurses, or the three-man carry from the room or removal to a wheeled stretcher might best serve the purpose, depending upon the number of nurses available.

41

A bed on fire should never be pulled out into a corridor, where drafts may increase the seriousness of the fire, and the sight of the fire by other patients may cause panic.

Some nurses have expressed alarm about the flammability of nylon. The main problem with nylon is that it is likely to cause an accumulation of static electricity. For this reason, nylon outer garments are taboo in areas in which anesthetics are used. The fact that nylon may cause an accumulation of static electricity does not, however, mean that it has unusual burning properties. In fact, it is rated at the bottom of a list of synthetic materials as far as ignition potential is concerned.

Wastebasket fires

Questions are often asked about handling wastebasket fires. It is pointed out that blankets and sheets are not available in office locations and that extinguishers are often some distance away. These fires can be put out by completely covering the top of the container with a magazine, or a newspaper. If nothing else is handy, a person can remove his suit coat, grasp a shoulder of the coat in each hand and drape it over the container.

Burning liquids and gases

When pressure or cylinder gases or liquids are burning, it is necessary to first shut off the source of supply. If this is not possible, adjacent materials, which are combustible or explosive, should be removed. A blazing cylinder might be wheeled or carted to a safer location; even outside.

Burning liquids and gases can be handled safely. For example, the pilot light on a gas range burns continuously, yet there is no danger unless the light goes out and fumes accumulate in the room. Then, however, ignition sources of any kind can be disastrous. Unless the supply of liquid or gas can be shut off, it might be wise to avoid extinguishment. Firemen have been killed because they extinguished gas meter fires in basements before the supply was cut off. Putting out a gaseous or liquid fuel fire while fumes are leaking or still running into the area can be fatal. The sudden re-ignition from the heat already present can blow a building apart. Burning gaseous or liquid fuel presents less of a danger potential than an "empty" fuel container (which actually contains exposive vapors) exposed to heat. This is true whether the container is a can, a cylinder, or a room.

FIRE FIGHTING EQUIPMENT

Portable fire extinguishers can often cope with gaseous-, liquid-, or solid-fuel fires in their early stages and prevent their spread. It is therefore necessary for all personnel to know how to operate the various kinds of extinguishers found in hospitals. There may be some hesitancy on the part of untrained personnel in using fire extinguishers. Such hesitancy can best be dispelled by demonstrations of the equipment and actual use of the equipment by personnel. Any mechanical device can be understood better if it is operated by those who will be expected to use it. There are several different kinds of extinguishers. Each is suitable for different locations and should be used only for the kind of fire for which it is designed. In general, the best pair of extinguishers for all patient areas and the best and easiest combination for women to use is the pressurized water (by air) extinguisher and the five pound carbon dioxide extinguisher. The label, or data plate on each extinguisher offers a ready reference and should be reviewed frequently during routine tours of duty so that its content is familiar *before* a fire emergency.

Stored-pressure water extinguishers

Stored-pressure water extinguishers are used for textile, wood, or rubbish fires. They are not to be used on fires involving oils or flammable liquids, or electrical equipment. Units are capable of continuous or intermittent operation.

Extinguishers should be located where temperatures do not exceed 120°F, nor go below 40°F. Antifreeze, usually inhibited calcium chloride, can be added if need be; check with the manufacturer of the extinguisher.

The single chamber of the unit contains both water and expellant gas. Pulling the locking pin and squeezing the combination handle operates the extinguisher. Do not put pressure on the discharge lever while removing the pin. The units will discharge a solid stream of water up to 30 or 40 feet horizontally. They can be operated while being carried.

To use, remove the extinguisher from its wall bracket by lifting with the carrying handle and the bottom lip. Carry it to the fire by the handle. Remove the locking pin. Squeeze the discharge lever and direct the water stream at the base of the flames; work from side to side or around the fire and as close to the fire as possible. After the flames are extinguished, direct the water at smouldering or glowing surfaces.

FIRE EXTINGUISHER/AGENT

SUITABLE FOR USE ON TYPE OF FIRE	AGENT CHARACTERISTICS	Available Sizes	Horizontal Range	Discharge Time
REGULAR OR ORDINARY DRY CHEMICAL ★				
B C	Basically Sodium Bicarbonate. Discharges a white cloud. Leaves residue. Non-freezing.	1 to 30 lbs.	5 to 20 ft.	8 to 25 Sec.
MULTIPURPOSE DRY CHEMICAL ★				
△ **B** C OR **B** C △ CAPABILITY	Basically Ammonium Phosphate. Discharges a yellow cloud. Leaves residue. Non-freezing. Some extinguishers utilizing this agent do not have an "A" rating — however, they are designated as having "A" capability.	2 to 30 lbs.	5 to 20 ft.	8 to 25 Sec.
PURPLE-K DRY CHEMICAL ★				
B C	Basically Potassium Bicarbonate. Discharges a bluish cloud. Leaves residue. Non-freezing.	2 to 30 lbs.	5 to 20 ft.	8 to 25 Sec.
KCL DRY CHEMICAL ★				
B C	Basically Potassium Chloride. Discharges a white cloud. Leaves residue. Non-freezing.	2 to 30 lbs.	5 to 20 ft.	8 to 25 Sec.
	Potassium Chloride/Urea	11 to 23	15 to 30	20 to 31
CARBON DIOXIDE				
B C	Basically an inert gas that discharges a cold white cloud. Leaves no residue. Non-freezing.	2½ to 20 lbs.	3 to 8 ft.	8 to 30 Sec.

★ NOTE: Available in stored pressure or cartridge operated types.

44

CHARACTERISTICS

SUITABLE FOR USE ON TYPE OF FIRE	AGENT CHARACTERISTICS	Available Sizes	Horizontal Range	Discharge Time
HALOGENATED AGENT				
B	Basically halogenated hydro-carbons. Discharges a white vapor. Leaves no residue. Non-freezing.	2½ lb.	4 to 8 ft.	.8 to 10 Sec.
WATER ▲				
A	Basically tap water. Discharges in a solid or spray stream. (May contain corrosion in-hibitor which leaves a yellow residue.) Protect from freezing!	2½ Gal.	30 to 40 ft.	1 Minute
ANTI-FREEZE SOLUTION				
A	Basically a Calcium Chloride solution to prevent freezing. Discharges a solid or spray stream. Leaves residue. Non-freezing.	2½ Gal.	30 to 40 ft.	1 Minute
LOADED STREAM				
A B	Basically an alkali-metal-salt solution to prevent freezing. Discharges a solid or spray stream. Leaves residue. Non-freezing.	2½ Gal.	30 to 40 ft.	1 Minute
FOAM				
B	Basically water and detergent. Discharges a foamy solution. After evaporation, leaves a powder residue. Protect from freezing.	18 oz.	10 to 15 ft.	24 Sec.
DRY POWDER SPECIAL COMPOUND				
D	Basically Sodium Chloride or Graphite materials. Agent is discharged from an extin-guisher in a solid stream or is applied with a scoop or shovel to smother combustible metal. Leaves residue. Non-freezing.	30 lbs.	5 to 20 ft.	25 to 30 Sec.

▲ NOTE: Pump tanks available.

Courtesy Fire Equipment Manufacturers' Association, Inc., Mt. Prospect, Ill. 60056.

45

Carbon dioxide (CO₂) extinguishers

A carbon dioxide (CO_2) extinguisher is used on fire involving oils, all flammable liquids, or electrical equipment. The extinguishers come in various sizes according to the weight of the carbon dioxide content. When the pin which locks the handles is pulled out, and the handles are pressed together, or the wheel valve turned, a cloud of CO_2 gas is discharged through the horn. The horn of the extinguisher should be pointed about eight inches to the side of the fire, the handles pressed, and the blanket of gas drawn over the fire. Expansion of the gas cools some of it to a solid known as carbon dioxide "snow" or "dry ice."

Dry chemical extinguishers

Dry chemical extinguishers consist of internally or externally mounted cartridges of carbon dioxide or nitrogen gas which, when the top is punctured or the cartridge valve opened, expels chemically processed bicarbonate of soda powder from the outer shell through the hose and nozzle. The inert gas and the chemical action of the powder will smother a fire. (For portable extinguishers, the range is 8 to 12 feet.)

Dry chemical units may be used on oil, grease, gasoline, and other solvent fires, and on electrical equipment fires. Dry chemical or dry powder extinguishers should be used for work areas where men are more likely to use them, such as boiler rooms, power plants, paint shops, and the like.

When an extinguisher is carried to a fire; the locking pin should be removed; and the dry chemical chamber pressured by puncturing the cartridge or opening the cartridge valve. (The discharge is controlled by squeezing the nozzle handle.)

Some hospitals, by choice or through fire department advice, have installed ABC multi-purpose extinguishers throughout all areas, exclusively. These extinguishers have little penetrating power, although they are good for surface fires. Using these types of extinguishers, will, for example, extinguish a small fire, however, it may smoulder and flare up again, unless it is removed and thoroughly wetted down.

Though there are multi-purpose extinguishers, they are compromises, and should not be used exclusively. (With these, as with all extinguishers, the local fire department should be consulted for professional advice on their use and placement.)

There is some controversy about the use of these extinguishers in patient areas, because of possible respiratory problems that may arise from airborne contaminants, after use.

Hose lines

If the fire cannot be subdued with one or two extinguishers, a hose line should be employed. A fire can be extinguished by turning on the water and moving the stream back and forth across the burning material. The amount of water received depends upon how much or how little the valve at the outlet is opened.

The hose is attached to a gate valve. The more the valve wheel is turned, the wider it opens the gate and the greater is the flow of water. It is exactly like opening a window. If one wants a little air, he opens the window a little. He may get more air than he cares for by opening the window wide. On the same principle, the valve wheel should be turned slowly.

A hose line is usually seventy-five or one hundred feet long. It requires three nurses to operate it, one at the valve wheel and one on each side of the hose just behind the nozzle. The flow of water through the hose pushes back on the persons holding the line; therefore, it must be held firmly. The nurses operating the hose should kneel in the doorway first, moving the stream up and down and side-to-side, while hitting the fire. In this position, the smoke and heat will pass harmlessly over their heads. The fire cannot be extinguished by washing flame and smoke. It is necessary to spray water on the actual material which is burning. When it is fairly dark in the room and the nurses can see more white steam than black smoke, they should stand up and move in to kill what little fire is left. When they are satisfied that the fire is extinguished, the water should be turned off.

To rid the room of smoke, the corridor door should be closed and the window or windows of the room opened ten inches from the top and ten inches from the bottom. By such action a change from foul to fresh air can be quickly accomplished. Debris should be closely inspected before being removed to avoid the possibility of rekindling.

If a great deal of smoke or heat prevents extinguishing the fire, the door to the room should be closed and a wet towel or blanket placed across the threshold. This will prevent the hot gases and the smoke from entering the hall or corridor. (It takes quite a while for fire to burn through a solid door.)

The next operation to consider is evacuation, which means moving all patients from the vicinity of the room just closed off. See pages 27 through 32.

Inverting-type extinguishers

Inverting-type fire extinguishers (soda-acid extinguishers and foam extinguishers) are no longer manufactured. They should be phased out of service.

Training Drills

The type of coordinated response described in the preceding sections is possible only if hospitals set up realistic fire emergency training programs that require the participation of all their staff in actual practice of the techniques of fire extinguishment and patient removal. These are skills one does not learn simply by reading about them or watching someone else demonstrate them.

Most of the hospitals that have initiated training programs work with only small groups at a time. This allows the training to proceed without disrupting the necessary routine. Often a nucleus of from six to twelve nurses or other personnel is trained first and they carry on the instructions. This original corps should probably not be burdened with training the whole hospital. They can, however, indoctrinate another group and then drop out. The second group can then train the third and so on.

Nurses have not only trained themselves but also trained male aids and orderlies. In many cases, a team trained at one hospital instructs personnel at another hospital.

One of the best methods of training is the use of drills. In setting up training drills, it is convenient to use three nurses to make the carries and three nurses dressed in slacks to act as patients. Light "patients" should be used at first until the nurses learn the removal mechanics. Then the poundage can be increased sharply, even to the point of using men as "patients."

Here is how some hospitals add realism to a training drill—they first make sure, however, that their local fire department permits it and will supervise it. Next, they select a training area that is well away from the patient area. Two or three metal scrub pails are placed about the training area and one or two ounces (or 25 to 50cc) of naphtha or white (unleaded) gasoline are placed in each pail. (They do not use benzene because it gives off a sooty smoke.) Each pail is set on fire by throwing in a lit match.

An alarm clock or bell can be used for the alarm. The nurses can use various carry combinations to remove the patients, either out a door or, for training purposes, behind a screen. On some drills the patient can be removed first and then the fires put out.

48

On other drills, the procedure can be reversed. Some fires should be put out with an extinguisher, and some with a piece of blanket or sheet about two feet square.

In mild weather, the beds can be set up out-of-doors in yards, courts, or driveways. Two small fires can be built near the beds and a larger fire some distance behind. These outside fires should be kindled from paper and wood. The larger fire should contain crates or lumber, but should have a back-stop to prevent the fire or debris from scattering.

The small fires can be put out with pressure or other suitable extinguishers, the large fires with the hose line. All the equipment should be explained and discussed and used by everyone present. An outside demonstration of this kind could be timed to fit in with the annual date of extinguisher recharge. Thus, a number of people can take educational advantage of something which has to be done anyway. It seems wasteful for one man to be delegated to dump a dozen extinguishers in a solitary task when so many others could benefit.

Practice in carrying "patients" on stairs and fire escapes is especially valuable, for it will help overcome any fear about working at heights and personnel will learn that they need not worry about synchronizing their walking with each other. It will follow naturally. To start with, it is usually best to work with volunteers. People who are forced to do something are harder to teach. In addition, it is safer for all concerned if the persons handling fires and weight and working at heights are interested in what they are doing.

It does no harm to inject a little humor into safety instruction. It is not necessary for a safety discourse to be as sombre as a funeral oration. Once, for example, when the author was describing a two-man removal to a large group of student nurses, he remarked that he usually had some big fat fellow play the patient, but as long as none was available he would have to do something else. There was a lull, as he expected, for a second or two. Then a voice in the back squealed, "How about you?" All the students applauded and cheered and even stamped their feet. It turned out to be a very good meeting.